*fit*SATIONAL

Daily Physical, Mental & Spiritual Fitness Tips

ANDREA GEORGE-CARRINGTON

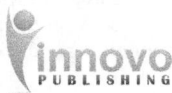

innovo
PUBLISHING

Published by Innovo Publishing, LLC
www.innovopublishing.com
1-888-546-2111

innovo
PUBLISHING

Publishing quality books, eBooks, audiobooks, music, screenplays & courses for the Christian & wholesome markets since 2008.

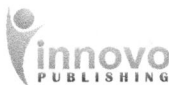

FITSATIONAL
Daily Physical, Mental & Spiritual Fitness Tips

Library of Congress Control Number: 2023923453
ISBN: 978-1-61314-974-4

Cover Design & Interior Layout: Innovo Publishing, LLC

Printed in the United States of America
U.S. Printing History
First Edition: 2023

Has God called you to create a Christ-centered or wholesome book, eBook, audiobook, music album, screenplay, or online course? Visit Innovo's educational center (cpportal.com) to learn how to accomplish your calling with excellence.

This book is dedicated to Pearl Robinson, my aunt, and Betty George, my mom: women with big hearts and strong vision, whose support of my interest in health and fitness as a child gave me the opportunity to experience the spiritual side of wellness. At an early age, they took me to the spa frequently and taught me the importance of eating healthy and presenting my body as the body of Christ.

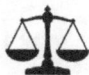

Introduction

Welcome to *Fitsational*—the book. What you will find in these pages is a combination of inspirational and spiritual health and fitness tips written to exercise your mind and your spirit. These tips will help you to develop physically, mentally, and emotionally, and teaches you how to develop your spiritual health as well.

Author Andrea George-Carrington is an educator, philosopher, teacher, instructor, and native Texan. With over forty-one years of experience in the health and fitness industry and her love for traveling around the world in search of more knowledge, her hundreds of successful fitness instructor clients speak of her wisdom in the field. She specializes in low-impact aerobics, water aerobics, kids fitness, senior adult programs, recreational activities, nutrition, minority health issues, and much more. Her focus is on safe, effective exercises. Andrea is the owner of Workouts by Andrea and The Fit Kids Corporation—a nonprofit health and fitness organization for kids. She previously owned Workouts by Andrea's Family Fitness Center, Aerobic Certification Company, and the Jr. Starz Basketball Association, and she is currently the founder and producer of *Fitsational*, the health and fitness exercise TV talk show, radio show (rejoice-now.com), and now, book.

As you read through this booklet, may you be challenged, encouraged, and strengthened by the truths of God's Word as it applies to your physical, mental, emotional, and spiritual health.

Twitter: @fitsational
Instagram: @thefitkidscorp
Podcast: https://www.podomatic.com/podcasts/workoutsbyandrea
Facebook @thefitkidscorp

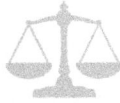

What God Has Written

*"And men shall speak of the might of thy terrible acts:
and I will declare thy greatness."*
—*Psalm 145:6*

The *cause* of all physical disease and mental malaise
[Satan] wants us to be ignorant of his devices and
how to defuse them.

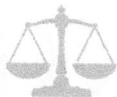

Health

Health is more than merely the absence of disease. Total well-being is a balance between all aspects of our lives: spiritual, physical, emotional, and mental.

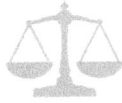

How to Develop Your Spiritual Health

"Like newborn babies [you should] long for the pure milk of the word, so that by it you may be nurtured and grow in respect to salvation [its ultimate fulfillment]."
—*1 Peter 2:2* AMP

"But have nothing to do with irreverent folklore and silly myths. On the other hand, discipline yourself for the purpose of godliness [keeping yourself spiritually fit]."
—*1 Timothy 4:7* AMP

"Praise ye the Lord: for it is good to sing praises unto our God; for it is pleasant; and praise is comely."
—*Psalm 147:1*

"Let every soul be subject unto the higher powers. For there is no power but of God: the powers that be are ordained of God."
—*Romans 13:1*

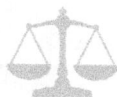

Discovering God's Purpose for Your Life

Recognize that God has a wonderful plan for your life.

"'For I know the plans and thoughts that I have for you,' says the Lord, 'plans for peace and well-being and not for disaster, to give you a future and a hope.'"
—Jeremiah 29:11 AMP

You will never fulfill God's purpose until there is a transformation of the mind.

"And do not be conformed to this world [any longer with its superficial values and customs], but be transformed and progressively changed [as you mature spiritually] by the renewing of your mind [focusing on godly values and ethical attitudes], so that you may prove [for yourselves] what the will of God is, that which is good and acceptable and perfect [in His plan and purpose for you]."
—Romans 12:2 AMP

"And we know that all things work together for good to them that love God, to them who are the called according to his purpose."
—Romans 8:28

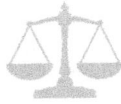

How to Become Spiritually, Mentally, Emotionally, and Physically Fit

"And let endurance have its perfect result and do a thorough work, so that you may be perfect and completely developed [in your faith], lacking in nothing."
—*James 1:4* AMP

"Trust in the Lord with all your heart and lean not on your own understanding; in all your ways submit to him, and he will make your paths straight."
—*Proverbs 3:5-6* NIV

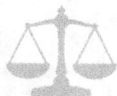

Get In Shape

S—*piritual*
H—*ealth*
A—*ttitude*
P—*urpose*
E—*conomics*

"Wherefore take unto you the whole armour of God, that ye may be able to withstand in the evil day, and having done all, to stand."
—*Ephesians 6:13*

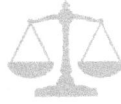

How to Glorify God with Your Body

"What? know ye not that your body is the temple of the Holy Ghost which is in you, which ye have of God, and ye are not your own? For ye are bought with a price: therefore glorify God in your body, and in your spirit, which are God's."
—1 Corinthians 6:19-20

Remember: your body was bought with a price. Be obligated to God, be disciplined, and yield not to temptation. God can take a nobody and make him/her into somebody.

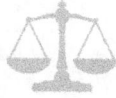

God's Dedication to Good Health

"Beloved, I wish above all things that thou mayest prosper and be in health, even as thy soul prospereth."
—*3 John 2*

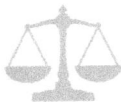

God's Health Plan for a Healthier Body, Mind, and Emotional State

God's love:

"Beloved, let us [unselfishly] love and seek the best for one another, for love is from God; and everyone who loves [others] is born of God and knows God [through personal experience]. The one who does not love has not become acquainted with God [does not and never did know Him], for God is love. [He is the originator of love, and it is an enduring attribute of His nature.]"
—1 John 4:7-8 AMP

"But God clearly shows and proves His own love for us, by the fact that while we were still sinners, Christ died for us."
—Romans 5:8 AMP

"And Jesus replied to him, '"YOU SHALL LOVE THE LORD YOUR GOD WITH ALL YOUR HEART, AND WITH ALL YOUR SOUL, AND WITH ALL YOUR MIND." This is the first and greatest commandment. The second is like it, "You shall love your neighbor as yourself [that is, unselfishly seek the best or higher good for others]."'"
—Matthew 22:37-39 AMP

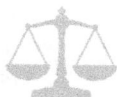

Emergency and Intensive Care

End waiting around.
"In my trouble I cried to the LORD, And He answered me."
—*Psalm 120:1* AMP

Often, God's nick-of-time surgery takes more than a few minutes, but even then, it can be a happy combination of the emergency room and the operating room in one convenient place and time period.

"Do not be anxious or worried about anything, but in everything [every circumstance and situation] by prayer and petition with thanksgiving, continue to make your [specific] requests known to God. And the peace of God [that peace which reassures the heart, that peace] which transcends all understanding, [that peace which] stands guard over your hearts and your minds in Christ Jesus [is yours]."
—*Philippians 4:6-7* AMP

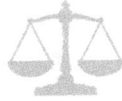

Creative Claim Services

How to file and get approval:
"You will also decide and decree a thing, and it will be established for you."
—Job 22:28 AMP

"And the very God of peace sanctify you wholly; and I pray God your whole spirit and soul and body be preserved blameless unto the coming of our Lord Jesus Christ."
—1 Thessalonians 5:23

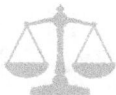

Wait to Lose Weight

*"But they that wait upon the L*ORD *shall renew their strength; they shall mount up with wings as eagles; they shall run, and not be weary; and they shall walk, and not faint."*
—*Isaiah 40:31*

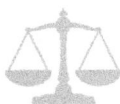

Spiritual Exercises

"So then faith cometh by hearing, and hearing by the word of God."
—Romans 10:17

Exercise your faith and build your spiritual muscle.
Speak aloud to yourself,
"[I will] resist the devil, and he will flee from [me]."
—James 4:7

I am a believer; therefore,
"In My name they will cast out demons."
—Mark 16:17 AMP

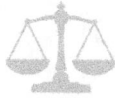

Walk for Your Health

"If we walk in the light, as he is in the light, we have fellowship one with another."
—1 John1:7

"I will walk among you, and will be your God, and ye shall be my people."
—Leviticus 26:12

"Yea, though I walk through the valley of the shadow of death, I will fear no evil: for thou art with me; thy rod and thy staff they comfort me."
—Psalm 23:4

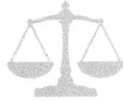

How to Exercise Your Authority

At the first sign of difficulty, confess: *spirit of pain, arthritis, indigestion, headache, discouragement, fear, anxiety, stress, resentment, anger, and rejection—I refuse you! In the name of Jesus.*

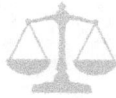

Believe in Yourself

Have faith in your abilities. Without a humble but reasonable confidence in your own powers, you cannot be successful or happy. But with sound self-confidence, you can succeed.

A sense of inferiority and inadequacy interferes with the attainment of your hopes, but self-confidence leads to self-realization and successful achievement.

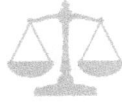

Have Faith

In your exercise program, remember that fitness is the intangible—it's the thing you cannot see. But,

"Faith is the substance of things hoped for, the evidence of things not seen."
—Hebrews 11:1

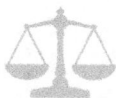

Procrastination

Do you procrastinate on God's exercise program?
Sometimes you work out, sometimes you don't?
Christ says,

*"So then because thou art lukewarm, and neither cold
nor hot, I will spue thee out of my mouth."*
—Revelation 3:16

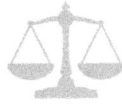

How to Draw upon that Higher Power

Learn to take a positive, optimistic attitude toward every problem. In direct proportion to the intensity of the faith that you muster, you will receive power to meet your situations.

"According to your faith be it unto you."
—*Matthew 9:29*

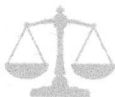

Adding Humor to Your Life

Maximize the things that make you laugh, and share humorous things with each other. Learn to anticipate trouble, and be prepared to face it with humor. Turn a negative situation into a positive one using humor.

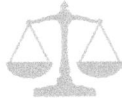

How to Have Constant Energy

How you *think* you feel has a dramatic effect on how you *actually* feel physically. If your mind tells you that you are tired, the body mechanism, the nerves, and the muscles accept the fact. If your mind is intensely interested, you can continue an activity indefinitely.

"In him we live, and move, and have our being."
—Acts 17:28

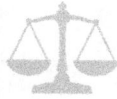

Stability

He is my rock, He is my fortress, He is my deliverer, He is my strength, He is my shield, He is the horn of my salvation, He is my power, He is my joy (of whom and what shall I be afraid?), He makes my way perfect, He is my stay. If God be for me, who can be against me? He is always present, He is my shepherd, He is my provider, He is my peace.

My times are made stable by His wisdom and knowledge. I am established in righteousness. Oppression, fear, and terror are far from me. I stay calm in the midst of strife, fear, anger, and other obstacles the enemy throws at me by attending to God's Word.

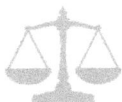

How to Meditate

Meditation is worshipping God in spirit and in truth.

God is Spirit:

"And they that worship him must worship him in spirit and in truth."
—John 4:24

"His delight is in the law of the Lord; and in his law doth he meditate day and night."
—Psalm 1:2

A quiet reflection upon the words of scripture:

"Thy testimonies are my meditation."
—Psalm 119:99

A prayerful review of scripture:

"Meditate upon these things."
—1 Timothy 4:15

"My meditation of him shall be sweet."
—Psalm 104:34

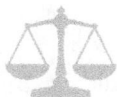

How to Use Faith in Healing

Remember that God does nothing except by law.

God has arranged two remedies for all illness:
one is healing through natural laws applicable by
science, and the other brings healing by spiritual law
applicable by faith.

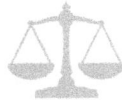

Inherited Diseases

Prune the family tree:

"Visiting (avenging) the iniquity (sin, guilt) of the fathers upon the children and the grandchildren to the third and fourth generations [that is, calling the children to account for the sins of their fathers]."
—*Exodus 34:7* AMP

God's laser surgery can root out any unhealthy residue passed on from ancestors to descendants by generational spirits.

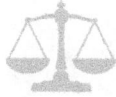

How to Defeat Fear

Confess,

"[I am a doer] of the word, and not [a hearer] only,
deceiving [my own self]."
—James 1:33

I am happy in those things that I do because I am a doer of the word of God.

I take the shield of faith and,

"Quench all the fiery darts of the wicked."
—Ephesians 6:16

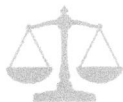

How to Defeat Worry and Fear

Confess,
"[I am] the body of Christ."
—1 Corinthians 12:27

Satan has no power over me, for I,
"Overcome evil with good."
—Romans 12:21

I am of God who has overcome Satan, for,
"Greater is he that is in [me], than he that is in the world."
—1 John 4:4

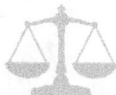

The Need for Pruning

"Every branch that does bear fruit he prunes so that it will be even more fruitful."
—John 15:2 NIV

Because our Father's heart is grieved each time we go astray, He lifts His chastening hand in love to guide us in His way. Christ the gardener cuts away the dead wood to make us fruitful.

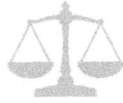

Bread and Butter

"With the measure you use, it will be measured to you."
—*Matthew 7:2* NIV

Don't be too hard on the person who sins, for the yardstick you lay on another may someday be used as a measure for you. Oh, be gracious and judge not my brother! The fault you see in another just might be your own.

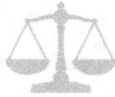

Physical Needs

*"Delight [yourself] in the LORD, and He will give [you]
the desires and petitions of [your] heart."*
—Psalm 37:4 AMP

With what measure I meet, it is measured unto me.

*"[I] soweth bountifully [and] shall reap also bountifully....
[I] give; not grudgingly, or of necessity: for God loveth
a cheerful giver.... [And I have] all sufficiency in all
things ... [to] abound to every good work."*
—2 Corinthians 9:6-8

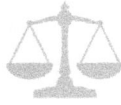

Believing

I give no place to the devil. Every principality, every power, every ruler of the darkness of this world, and every wicked spirit in the heavenly places must bow its knee to the name of Jesus. Jesus is the Lord of my body. He is the Lord of finances. Jesus is the Lord of my life!

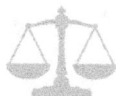

How to Obtain Wisdom and Guidance

"The Spirit of truth, is come, he will guide [me] into all truth."
—John 16:13

I have perfect knowledge of every situation and every circumstance that I come up against, for I have the wisdom of God. Therefore, I confess,

"If [I] lack wisdom, let [me] ask of God, that giveth to all men liberally, and upbraideth not; and it shall be given [me]."
—James 1:5

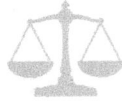

How to Overcome Arthritis

Confess by faith, *I believe that I can be healed right now of arthritis because,*

"Greater is he that is in [me], than he that is in the world."
—*1 John 4:4*

I believe that God's Word is alive and full of power: acting, operating, energizing, and effective.

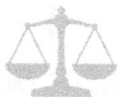

God's Personal Instructions for Relieving Stress

"But thou, O man of God, flee these things; and follow after righteousness, godliness, faith, love, patience, meekness. Fight the good fight of faith, lay hold on eternal life, whereunto thou art also called, and hast professed a good profession before many witnesses."
—1 Timothy 6:11-12

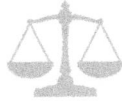

To Love

I am a new creature in love. My spirit is created in the image of love, and the Holy Spirit teaches me to love as He loves; therefore, I can never fail.

"Love is patient, love is kind. . . . Love never fails."
—1 Corinthians 13:4-8 NIV

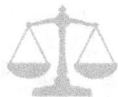

To Smile

A smile is the quickest way to combat the blues and connect you to other people. Add a little nonsense to your daily routine to liven it up and let go of your problems and disappointments quickly.

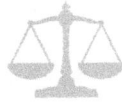

Overeating and Overindulging

Are you an overeater, or do you have a tendency to overindulge and need a little spiritual help? Confess, *I am an overcomer:*

"[I] overc[o]me him by the blood of the Lamb, and by the word of [my] testimony."
—Revelation 12:11

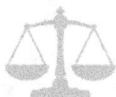

How to Become One of the Strongest People Alive

"God is my strength and power: and he maketh my way perfect."
—2 Samuel 22:33

You may not be the strongest or greatest. Your presence may not even count at all. But when you put your trust in Jesus' power, you can be assured He'll never let you fall.

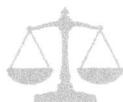

How to Have Harmony in Your Home

A home can be a special place of refuge, surrounding you with peace and precious things.

"Through wisdom is an house builded; and by understanding it is established."
—Proverbs 24:3

Skillful and godly wisdom is a house, a life, a home, and a family built, and then by good understanding it is established on a good foundation.

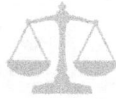

A Prayer for the Children

I pray that the children are disciples taught of the Lord and obedient to Your will. Great is their peace and undisturbed composure. I believe we receive wisdom and counsel in bringing up our children in the discipline and true yield of the Lord, and Your Word declares that when they are old, they will not depart from it. So I commit them into Your keeping, and I know and have confidence and trust that they are watched over and blessed of the Lord all the days of their lives. In Jesus' name, amen.

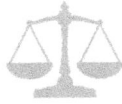

Fitness Training

"Train up a child in the way he should go: and when he is old, he will not depart from it."
—Proverbs 22:6

And teach your child how important it is to have friends that are in Christ.

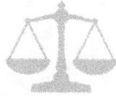

God's Exercise Program

"Confess [y]our sins."
—1 John 1:9

"Keep his commandments."
—1 John 2:3

"Walk, even as he walked."
—1 John 2:6

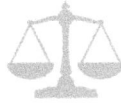

Healing for the Land

"If my people, which are called by my name, shall humble themselves, and pray, and seek my face, and turn from their wicked ways; then will I hear from heaven, and will forgive their sin, and will heal their land. Now mine eyes shall be open, and mine ears attent unto the prayer that is made in this place."
—2 Chronicles 7:14-15

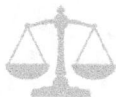

A Prayer for the Body of Christ

"For this cause I bow my knees unto the Father of our Lord Jesus Christ, of whom the whole family in heaven and earth is named, that he would grant you, according to the riches of his glory, to be strengthened with might by his Spirit in the inner man."
—Ephesians 3:14-16